THE TRUE SECRET
TO WEIGHT LOSS
IS *ENERGY*

How to Forget about Dieting,
Restore Your Natural Energy, and
Attain Your Ideal Weight

Randy Colton Rolfe

Ambassador Family Press
West Chester, PA

The True Secret to Weight Loss Is *Energy*

Copyright © 2012 Randy Colton Rolfe

ISBN-13:978-1477605974
ISBN-10:1477605975

Ambassador Family Press
West Chester, PA

CONTENTS

PREFACE

After forty years of teaching and practicing good nutrition, family wellness, and total health, I have here condensed all that I know to be true about weight loss. My remarks are based on personal experience, family experience, years of study, success with hundreds of clients, examination of the scientific research, investigation of human history and ancestry, close observation of current cultural conditions and issues, and common sense.

In these eighteen short chapters, I hope you will find the answers you seek. You will feel renewed hope that you can achieve your ideal weight comfortably and permanently. And you can move forward quickly to your goals with confidence and excitement.

In 2010, 60% of Americans were overweight, and over half of those were obese. That means 60% have a Body Mass Index of 25 or more, and 35% have a BMI of 30 or more. Between 18.5 and 24.9 is the healthiest range to minimize heart disease, stroke, certain cancers, type 2 diabetes, and other problems. In 2000, no states had 30% obese. Yet by 2010, 12 states had 30% obese, and even Colorado, the slimmest state, had 20% obese. The Centers for Disease Control and Prevention report that $147 billion a year in medical costs are attributable to obesity. We all know to eat less and exercise more. Why don't we?

You will discover that putting on extra weight is seldom about being lazy, gluttonous, dumb, ignorant, or uncaring about your health or appearance. It is most often about serious misinformation about how our bodies and minds work and how our food and lifestyle habits affect us. In this book you will find out exactly how to make small incremental changes over the next few days and weeks which can change your life for the better before you know it.

Of necessity I will be speaking in generalities, so nothing in this book can or should replace professional advice from your own personal health care advisers. Nevertheless, the information in this little book can transform your body and mind. Simple, easy steps that make sense to you will invigorate your efforts to be the person you want to be.

CHAPTER 1

IT'S NOT JUST ABOUT EAT LESS, EXERCISE MORE

Certainly the scientific numbers tell you that if you are overweight, you are taking in more calories than you are using, so that your body stores away extra calories in fat. So it seems like the scientific answer is to eat less and exercise more. Doctors often say that this is the simple secret. But millions try to do this every day and it doesn't seem to be working. Billions of dollars are spend every week on ways to help people lose weight and yet our population gets heavier and heavier, at younger and younger ages. What's going wrong?

If we were machines which could be programmed by pressing a few buttons, this advice might work. Press the button for less food in and the button for more exercise and the changes will happen. But thankfully we are not machines. We are living, feeling, loving creatures. We don't act from science. We act first from our survival instincts, and our decisions based on reasoning and science come only as a distant second.

But fifty years ago, most Americans were thin. Our instincts kept our waists small. What has happened in the last fifty years that has resulted in almost half our population going from being a healthy weight to being an unhealthy weight? It is no surprise that several factors have come together to make such a huge change in a whole population in such a short time.

First, when we eat a typical American diet today, we miss the micronutrients which are no longer there. Our bodies crave these micronutrients which are essential to our body processes, so we just keep eating more expecting to find them. For example, consider a slice of bread. Your body doesn't know that something that looks, smells, and tastes like a hearty grain product no longer has the proteins, oils, vitamins, minerals, and enzymes that it would have had a thousand years ago. It's the same with a strawberry flavored soda. You get the sweetness and flavor, but your body still looks for the vitamins, minerals, and so on which would have been in real strawberries. So without realizing it, you tend to just eat more and more, looking for the missing components.

Second, our lives have become far more complex and busy, with more irregular schedules, more demands coming from more different directions every day, multi-tasking expected of everyone, much more complicated family and household relationships, and ever increasing economic pressure on all but the very rich. All these factors mean daily and perpetual stress, which changes the way our bodies relate to food. Stress runs down our energy so we eat to get a quick energy boost. Stress changes our hormones so that more fat is stored. And when everything else is stressful, eating can become a distraction and a temporary escape, perhaps one of our few daily pleasures.

These are not the reasons you hear in the halls of policy or science. Our politicians and scientists are dependent on the larger economy, which is dependent on industry and profits. Food production is the same. The food production system makes more money from fabricated, processed foods than from organically grown fresh produce. Industry never looks back. It really doesn't care about how it was fifty or a thousand years ago, because it can't duplicate it. But our bodies do care. So we are caught between an ever poorer quality food mix and an ever more stressful lifestyle. As a consequence, we are a population suffering from ever increasing obesity.

What our popular culture and many of our policy makers, scientists, and health advisers tell us is that we lack will power, need to be more rational about what we consume, curb our appetite, stop the junk food, buy the healthy foods, end our hang-ups, get medical treatment for our disorders, get more fiber and water, or just stop being lazy, start moving, and get off our butts. The truth is we all hear these things every day. And Americans aren't stupid or uninformed. On the contrary, we are almost too plugged in. We hear such a constant barrage of misinformation about weight and how to lose it that we start to believe it.

Weight loss is not just about "eat less, exercise more." And it is not about will power, keeping count of calories or carbohydrates or fat. It's not about a too hefty appetite, too much junk food, or not enough healthy foods. It's not about a psychological hang-up or hormonal or metabolic imbalances. It's not about needing more fiber or water, or not getting enough exercise. All of these are involved in weight gain, but the secret to losing weight is energy.

If none of these are the true secret to weight loss, this means that even if you have a weight issue, you don't have to think of yourself as weak-willed, arithmetically challenged because you aren't counting, dumb for wanting junk foods, ignorant for not choosing healthier foods, saddled with an out of control appetite, marred by a psychological impediment, stuck with a physiological handicap, unaware of when you are thirsty, or just too lazy. You are none of these things. The true secret to weight loss is energy. Let me show you how.

CHAPTER 2
IT'S NOT ABOUT WILL POWER OR KEEPING COUNT

Will power is a mental exertion to overcome temptations of various kinds. It takes will power to run from a challenge, to avoid procrastination, to manage your temper, or to resist a thoughtless word or deed. But will power is not meant to counteract basic survival instincts like hunger, thirst, sleep, or the desire for human contact. People who "eat too much" don't lack will power. They lack the energy which the food, any kind of food, will give them.

Their will power will never be strong enough to counteract the survival instinct to do what it takes to get the energy to continue to function. Will power involves left brain activity or the super ego. It involves a judgment, that I should not eat this thing I want. It will lose out more often than not to the powerful right brain or limbic brain whenever it feels low on energy and cries out for food.

Keeping count is also a left brain activity. Counting, whether it's counting calories, carbs, fats, proteins, fiber, or ounces of water, will never give you the power to overcome the tastes, smells, textures, and boosts of energy that your right brain knows you will get from putting food in your mouth. Millions of people keep diaries of their foods, keep count of their daily intake of any number of things, make endless lists, refer to charts and columns of values, and wonder why they don't lose more weight or keep it off when they do lose some.

It's because eating is a right brain activity. It is a basic survival urge which no amount of will power or counting can negate.

There are many weight loss plans which have the personal touch. They have you visit a center, weigh in, chat with an expert counselor, review your records for the week, perhaps take classes, and get a pep talk. And every women's magazine has articles about one plan or another which promises to tell you what to eat at each meal so that the weight will come off. Yet these articles and programs just keep coming. If they worked, the support group plans and magazines would have to focus on something else.

Now there is actually a whole new industry developing. These programs advertise heavily. They not only plan your meals for you but deliver them to your door fully prepared. If these plans worked, why would our population be growing ever fatter and fatter?

Weight loss is not about will power or keeping count of various food components consumed. Don't let anyone shame you about this and don't shame yourself about it either.

CHAPTER 3
IT'S NOT ABOUT GLUTTONY, JUNK FOODS, OR HEALTH FOODS

Billions of dollars are spent every year to "suppress" the appetite. It is assumed we eat because our appetite tells us we are hungry. But most people I have helped who were overweight had no idea what feeling hungry feels like. Their appetite wasn't the problem. It was not their appetite which made them eat. They rarely fit the picture of the gluttonous overeaters. In fact, they were often stymied by how they couldn't lose weight even when they felt they were eating modestly and were serious about eating less. What got in their way was that dragging feeling. They mistook having low energy for being hungry. They ate not because they had a huge appetite but because they needed an energy boost.

Hunger is a feeling of emptiness in the stomach and gut which really only comes after you have been without food for many hours. One meal a day of balanced energy-building food can be enough to stave off any feeling of hunger. If everything in our bodies is working as it should, our livers have a wonderful storage function to measure out glucose as we need it. Among traditional tribal peoples, visitors have been astonished how they can go many hours, while hunting or migrating, without any need to eat. The fact that so many "diet" programs recommend five or six meals a day just goes to show that it is the drop in energy, not hunger or appetite, which moves people to eat.

Losing weight is not about ending our junk food habits either. Junk food gives us the energy lift we crave. Junk food gets made and eaten because food processors have found inexpensive ways to extract and concentrate all those food elements which give you the energy you seek. They have found ways to duplicate the tastes, smells, and textures which millions of years have taught your body to interpret as standing for good energy. So our junk foods give us big jolts of concentrated sugar, refined carbohydrates, fats, or all three. And there is usually added salt, to make us want more food or drink to dilute these elements for our metabolic processing. If we didn't crave the energy jolt, we wouldn't bother with the junk foods. If we had all the energy we wanted, we would be off doing more fun and active things with our bodies and minds. Avoiding junk foods isn't the secret to weight loss.

Weight loss isn't about eating more healthy foods either. It's about having enough on-going daily energy that junk foods don't tempt us. It is true that eating predominantly healthy foods helps you to get the energy you want each day. We will talk more about that later. But when you don't have the energy you need, what is going to give you the motivation to start eating healthy when the energy you need right now is readily available from a soda, a donut, or a latte?

CHAPTER 4
IT'S NOT ABOUT HANG-UPS OR DISORDERS

Much recent research has focused on the psychological and emotional aspects of eating disorders, such as excessive eating, anorexia, bulimia, carbohydrate addiction, sugar zombies, malnutrition through excessive alcohol consumption, and more. Certain habits and assumptions we pick up as children from our parents, teachers, schools, churches, neighbors, music lyrics, or TV can certainly start us off on the wrong track. In the highly stressed lifestyles of most families today, eating behaviors, like eating or not eating, being picky or not, and obeying dietary advice or not, form one of the few categories over which children have personal control. So psychologists observe that the children may get into the habit of using these behaviors to express themselves and to carve out a small but real domain where they do have control.

Many of these problems were much more unusual fifty years ago. As a parenting specialist, I can't help but notice that these problems became more common when parents had less and less time with their children. In the last twenty years, when both obesity and other eating disorders sky-rocketed, it has become rare for a parent to be around their children enough to be setting a good example of eating three "square" meals a day at regular intervals, with "no snacks between meals," and no desserts until dinner is finished. In many cases, bad habits evolved simply because no one was actually on the scene to instruct and guide otherwise.

This kind of history can be a strong negative factor in a person's efforts to achieve a healthy weight. But the bottom line is still a lack of energy. Accumulated bad habits can sabotage your body's natural ability to generate enough energy. Without that energy you don't feel good enough and strong enough to make healthy choices for yourself now. Persistent emotional hang-ups and bad habits and attitudes around food can certainly make losing weight harder, but they are not the key to the solution. We must first restore the body's natural energy. This will be the key to overcoming these bad habits and emotional issues.

In addition to looking at emotional aspects of weight control, recent science has focused on a cluster of physical conditions which occur when a person struggles with persistent extra weight. Chief among these are hormonal imbalance and what has come to be named metabolic syndrome. These disorders are more descriptive than explanatory of what's going on. Hormonal imbalance most commonly involves a sluggish thyroid. A sluggish thyroid means that the body cells produce energy slower than normal, because the thyroid gland controls the rate of metabolism in the cells. When the thyroid is not producing enough thyroid hormone to instruct the cells to turn up the heat, we feel fatigued and tired and find it harder to concentrate, focus, or make decisions. And if the cells are metabolizing slowly, the fuel which we have consumed from our food but is not getting used at a normal rate will be stored away as fat.

Metabolic syndrome is a recent diagnosis to explain persistent weight gain. Fat is stored primarily around the waist and upper body in this condition. Also blood sugar and fat balance are disturbed, usually as a result of decreased cellular responsiveness to the body's natural insulin. When carbohydrates are processed and refined, most of the fiber, oils, and protein have been removed, so they require little digestion. Refined carbohydrates can go quickly into the blood. The body is careful to maintain a steady blood sugar because the concentration of sugar in the blood affects whether each cell in the body is properly supplied. So any rise in blood sugar normally triggers production of insulin by the pancreas gland, and the insulin instructs the cells to pull in sugars from the blood.

If the body is repeatedly and chronically overloaded with too much carbohydrate time after time, the pancreas can fail to produce enough insulin at the right times. This causes blood sugar to get too high. Or the cells can become resistant to the effects of insulin. This also results in blood sugar getting too high. If the cells aren't taking in the sugar, energy isn't produced.

So again it is a lack of energy which makes the person eat more than their body theoretically needs to continue to function. Whether the pancreas is not producing enough insulin or the cells are resistant to it, in either case the cells are not getting the message to beef up their energy production. So the person feels run down and fatigued and their instincts tell them to rev up the fuel supply, by eating more.

Fortunately this situation is often reversible by using the measures we will be looking at shortly. So you don't need to feel that a diagnosis of hormonal imbalance or metabolic syndrome is a life sentence. Taking care to start normal energy production again can move you towards a better weight, reduce the metabolic imbalances, and have you feeling better.

CHAPTER 5
IT'S NOT ABOUT WATER, FIBER, OR BEING LAZY

We are often led to believe that someone struggling with their weight should just drink water when they get a snack attack or eat more high fiber foods so that their food digests more slowly and fills their stomach longer. Or we are led to believe that they're just too lazy to burn off the calories by getting moving. These are yet another set of myths.

The need for more fiber and pure water in the case of those struggling to lose weight cannot be denied, but it is not the cause of the weight problem. We have natural thirst urges and also a natural desire to chew hearty, textured foods. These food factors, fiber and water, are indeed the first things to go when foods are processed. But again it is not because people don't seek these out that they struggle with their weight. It is because these people lack energy.

When they are thirsty, they reach not for pure water but for a sugary drink, or at least a drink that tastes like sugar, because they are looking for energy. Likewise, chewing takes energy, and a candy bar low in fiber will give a whole lot more energy per chew than a bowl of oatmeal or a piece of whole wheat toast with real strawberry jam.

A vicious circle begins when a person has excess weight. Because of more tissue to take care of, the body has less energy left over for physical and mental activity, and less energy even for the digestive processes required to handle the extra food, especially the more concentrated foods of today. This situation can lead to poor digestion and poor absorption of food in the gut, which then can result in a number of problems, such as reflux of acids related to digestion, compaction in the digestive tract, and various immune responses, including irritable bowel symptoms and generalized low levels of inflammation throughout the body. These conditions can further drain the person's energy and make them want the quick fix of more food, rather than the "shoulds" of more water and fiber. So the secret to weight loss is not starting to consume more water and fiber. The secret is creating more energy, so that water and fiber are attractive again.

Sometimes people who are trying to lose weight hear that they need more water and start drinking huge amounts, thinking it will reduce their urge to eat or flush out toxins or increase metabolism. Often thirst can be interpreted as hunger and a glass of good water a little while before you eat can help to moderate your eating. But too much water or the wrong kind can actually sabotage your efforts. Much tap water and bottled water is highly acidic and often devoid of minerals. This means it will be an added stress on your body and can actually pull necessary minerals from your tissues. This can result in metabolic imbalances rather than in the healthy balance necessary to create healthy weight loss. It is important to keep your tissues properly hydrated, but alkaline, mineralized, energized water in moderation is what will assist you in losing weight. Drinking more water is not the key to weight loss.

The key to weight loss is not more exercise either. People are not as lazy as we are led to believe. We talk about couch potatoes, and we worry about kids who are glued to the screen. But I have yet to meet a child with normal energy levels who would not prefer to be running around outside with friends chasing birds and playing with sticks to sitting in front of a TV all day. It is only those children who lack energy who choose the couch. Again we have a vicious circle where extra weight makes people tired. But the solution is to up the energy level, not to pull them off the couch.

Which came first, the couch or the potato? I believe that it was the potato. The couch is only attractive because of the lack of energy and the already expanding waistline. And it was most likely lack of energy in the first place which led to the expanding waistline.

So now let's see how we can get that energy we need to get to our healthy weight.

CHAPTER 6
IT'S ALL ABOUT ENERGY

The problem of weight gain is so hard to solve because we look in all the wrong places for a solution. To build will power, we focus on instructions, plans, accountability, or a buddy system. To improve counting, we analyze every food, we try to live according to charts and plans, and we join support groups to compare notes. We argue about whether to count calories or carbs, fats or cholesterol. But we keep counting, even though history shows that most people who count end up losing and gaining repeatedly, often called the yo-yo diet plan.

We rail against all the junk foods, scare people with the piles of sugar in a soda or the amount of fat in a fried chicken wing, but these continue to sell even faster than ever. We pontificate endlessly on how easy it is to choose and prepare healthy foods, fresh produce, organic dairy and meats, and unprocessed, unpackaged foodstuffs. Yet those seeking to lose weight aren't usually the ones you see in the health food store.

We have endless appetite suppressants and medications to increase the sense of being full, to stimulate energy production, and to give us a quick shot of energy. With all the coffee shops serving up caffeine, the move to embrace chocolate for health and energy stimulation, and to give "five hour energy," are any of the folks embracing these solutions actually losing weight? No, because losing weight is about the natural production of energy at the cellular level.

We look to support groups and psychological help to overcome childhood abuse and neglect in order to help with weight control. These are very valuable and important for our overall well-being, but whether the weight problem is resolved by healing from these wrongs is another question.

For over 25 years I have been sharing with my students, clients, and audiences that obesity is a risk factor in itself for every major degenerative condition which currently plagues the developed countries. These include diabetes, cancer, auto-immune disorders, stroke, heart attack, and other problems as well. Now the medical world has come to see it that way too. But still doctors find it hard to get patients to lose weight once they have gained it. Instead they tend to resort to manipulating other key risk factors through medications or dietary restrictions.

As a result we are becoming a nation of folks who think they need medications to stay free of these debilitating diseases. In many cases, reducing weight would be the most effective and safest way to greatly reduce your chances of getting any of these diseases.

In a recent article in the *Journal of the American Medical Association*, the researchers found that between 2005 and 2010, only 1.2% of Americans engaged in the seven behaviors believed best to prevent cardiovascular disease. As bad as this sounds, this was down significantly from the 2% who covered these bases back in 1988 to 1994.

The seven behaviors are: not smoking, being physically active, having normal blood pressure, having healthy blood glucose levels, having healthy blood cholesterol levels, having a healthy weight, and following a healthy, balanced diet.

When an individual is overweight, each one of these factors takes a turn for the worse, except for the not smoking factor. With overweight and obesity on the rise, as well as the amount of money, media, and medicine spent on the problem, we are obviously barking up the wrong tree.

The true secret to weight loss is to help the body create the energy it needs not only to keep the body alive but also to make you actually feel good. You need to actually feel like moving your body. You need to feel like eating well. You need to feel like skipping a junky snack in favor of a walk, a talk with a friend, or a stab at the next work project. You need to feel good about yourself, who you are, and who you are becoming. To feel that way, you need to restore your natural energy.

So how do we help our bodies create this energy? It must come at the cellular level. Each organ in our bodies must be able to do its job for us to really feel good, what I call "vibrant health."

The brain needs to have lots of oxygen and glucose to feel good. That means the lungs must have energy to get the oxygen from the air, and the blood must have energy to move the oxygen and glucose to the brain. All the digestive organs must have energy to digest sugars and carbs to provide the glucose and to get all the other building blocks which brain tissue needs to be able to use the oxygen and glucose. The liver must have energy to process and store the glucose. The kidneys, hormones, and nerves need energy to regulate the movement of all the substances all these tissues need to do their work. The immune system and lymph system need energy to cleanse and protect the other organs from the wastes which can build up and from the useless chemicals which get into our bodies from our food and environment.

So the key is to get the energy production happening in every cell. But how do we do this? This will be the focus of the rest of this book.

CHAPTER 7
MORE ENERGY – WHERE TO START

What's the first thing a person disturbed by their weight notices about themselves? It's usually the waistline. We store fat on our tummies, especially if we are feeling any chronic stress. This is because cortisol, a stress-related hormone, causes the body to store away fat on the tummy. Depending on body type, different people store fat predominantly on different parts of the body, as we will see a bit later. But still, just about everyone will notice an increase in the waistline early on in the process of gaining weight.

The place to start for helping your body to create more natural energy is to improve your digestion. Isn't it nice that the first step to creating more energy in your body at the cellular level also will show quick results at the waistline?

People don't often think of improving digestion as the way to lose weight, but it is definitely the best first step to healthy weight loss. Here's why. People who are eating too many calories for the size of their body are overwhelming their digestive capacity. It is simple mechanics. There is too much food for that sized body to process it effectively.

It reminds me of my garbage disposal. I often put a banana skin down the disposal. I love bananas. But when making a fruit salad a few weeks ago, I skinned five bananas, and put them all down the disposal at once. Guess what happened? The disposal couldn't handle it. It failed.

So it is with a digestive system which is overwhelmed day after day with too much food. Our stomachs stretch, certainly, but our digestive organs can't keep putting out the extra enzymes and digestive acids necessary to process a whole lot of extra food, day after day. So what happens?

A cascade of unwanted effects follows. Undigested food sets up an environment for gas production by fermentative microbes in the gut. Burping and farting are the result. This undigested food can also cause irritation of the bowel lining, the leaking of pathogens and allergens into the blood stream from the digestive tract, and compaction in the lower intestine. Meanwhile, the digestive organs like the stomach, pancreas, small intestine, and gall bladder wear down. They may even produce fewer enzymes than they would normally with food intake at a workable level.

You end up with a lot of food going into fat storage. Meanwhile, the immune system, liver, and hormones are working overtime to control the effects on the blood system from this imbalanced process of digestion. Since every cell in the body is dependent on the right mix of nutrients and oxygen coming to it in the blood, the body takes great care to protect the balance of blood chemicals. When blood tests show that the fat, glucose, mineral, or vitamin levels are out of balance, either excessive or insufficient, you know that the digestive system already isn't working as well as it should.

To get cells producing the energy you deserve to have for body and mind, the digestive system must be protected.

CHAPTER 8
MORE ENERGY BY REBUILDING DIGESTION

So how do you rebuild a healthy digestive system? It may seem that the answer is just to eat less. But many people trying to lose weight already are eating way less than you think. This is because their systems have already slowed down under the burden of taking care of extra fat cells and dealing with the toxins from imbalanced metabolism. They are already feeling low on energy, so asking them to eat less to allow their digestion to rebuild is not likely to be successful.

The most effective way to rebuild the digestion for a person who wants to lose weight is to supplement the output of digestive enzymes and acids, known together as digestive juices. This breaks the cycle of degeneration. It must be kept in mind that the pancreas, stomach, gall bladder, and intestines are organs just like all the others in our bodies. They are made of cells which need nourishment. So there is a descending spiral of inefficiency if they do not produce what is needed to finish digestion properly. If the digestive juices they produce do not digest the food, then not only the other organs go without all the building blocks and fuel they need, but so do the digestive organs. So then they are even less able to produce their products to digest the next meal.

As living creatures, our energy comes from the earth, the sun, and our food and water. To create energy in our cells, we need fuel and oxygen, just like any candle. We get our oxygen mostly from the air we breathe, and it needs to be in a particular mix so that the pressure in our lungs and blood is maintained. As mammals, we cannot directly make our own fuel from sun, air, and soil like plants do. We depend on other life forms for our fuel. So we must eat these other life forms. These we call food. If it is not poisonous, we can eat it and get all the building blocks and fuel we need to nourish our cells.

As popular reporter and food enthusiast Michael Pollan has said, "Eat food, not too much, mostly plants." If we all followed this simple plan, most processed and packaged "foods" would be left off the plate because they also contain substances that are not foods. These are what Pollan calls "food like substances," or FLS. There are over 3,000 common additives which are not foods but which are added to our foods for different special effects. These are well described elsewhere. The point is, our digestive systems are stressed and sorely taxed to deal with them. Adding some digestive juices to start a better handling of our food can increase cellular energy production. It can also ease the burden on your digestion even before there is any reduction in total food.

When we develop in our mother's womb, we start out as a tube. The outside surface ends up as our skin and the inside surface ends up as our digestive system and lungs. These are the major interfaces with the outside world. What we put in our mouths must go through that long tube and have all the things we need sucked out of it and processed before it leaves our bodies at the other end. It's an awesome process which we should support. So let's look at how.

CHAPTER 9
MORE ENERGY FROM BETTER DIGESTIVE JUICES

The way to supplement your digestive juices so that your digestive system can get back on track is to eat supplements which contain digestive enzymes and digestive acids. You will need enzymes which digest four different categories of food: carbohydrates (including sugar, starch, and milk sugar), soluble fibers, fats, and proteins. You will also need betaine hydrochloride, which is the equivalent of the digestive acid which the stomach produces to break down fiber and protein.

I talk about "eating" supplements because it is important to realize that they are food. We sometimes "take" medications, which are alien substances designed to manipulate body processes to achieve a specific result in an acute situation. But we should "eat" our vitamins, minerals, and other supplements, because they are food. All pills are not the same.

Many people are apprehensive about adding acid when they already have reflux, where some of the acid content from the stomach returns in their esophagus when they eat aromatic foods like peppers or eat more than a small meal. But this result is usually because of not enough digestive acid in the stomach instead of too much.

The stomach is not producing enough acid at meal time due to stress or just too much food or the wrong mix of food. So fermentation happens, producing gas, which then must go either up or down. If it goes up it takes with it some mild acid from the stomach, which nevertheless can hurt since the esophagus is not designed for any acid. It can also carry up with it odors or tastes from the food in the stomach, such as from a green pepper. If the gas goes down instead, it causes unpleasant gas in the gut, bloating, and uncomfortable, smelly, and embarrassing release of intestinal gas.

Once I have explained this process to a client, they are willing to try the added stomach acid and are often amazed at its effectiveness. It can end reflux often immediately. It also prevents bloating and gassiness after a meal and helps to prevent gas in the lower bowel.

The enzymes which you eat should be sourced as much as possible from natural food sources. Many supplements on the market, for example, include bromelain which comes from pineapples. Other common foods with natural digestive properties are papaya and kiwifruit. Many raw foods contain some enzymes which help in the digestive process. But junk foods and all cooked and processed foods will contain none of these.

Studies have shown that it is hard to become seriously overweight if you are eating a largely raw, whole foods diet. It has also been demonstrated that when healthy children are presented with an array of natural, raw, whole foods, they tend to eat a completely balanced diet over the course of a week. It doesn't matter whether they are snacking, sitting down to eat, eating just one kind of thing all day and a different one the next day, or engaging in other patterns we tend to consider bad habits. This result shows that our natural appetites serve us well as long as they are not distorted by frequent consumption of processed, denatured foods.

So experience and science indicate that we must avoid overwhelming our digestive systems with foods which contain no live enzymes and are so processed and concentrated that they tax the digestive juices we do produce. If we avoid overwhelming our digestion, we are less likely to put on weight or to hold on to our extra weight. When our foods are properly digested, we get the energy we need at the cellular level to behave in healthier ways. We will be drawn to a more balanced diet and to healthier choices. We will feel like continuing to nurture a healthy digestive system and to create an upward spiral of health.

You can begin with a high quality digestive enzyme and acid combination, eating it just before or with your largest meal of the day. After a few days, eat one with each meal. Soon your digestion will feel a whole lot smoother and more complete. Bowel habits might change, food cravings might change, moods might improve, and your feeling of energy and get up and go will almost certainly improve.

Be sure not to dilute your digestive juices too much. Many people who are trying to lose weight are drinking all kinds of fluids in hopes of reducing their eating. But when you drink a lot of coffee, sodas, teas, or water near meal time, your digestive system has a hard time interpreting what juices are needed and also a hard time producing the juices which are needed. Don't drink more than eight ounces with a meal. And don't drink other liquids for at least two to three hours after a meal. Otherwise you will be diluting your digestive juices in the middle of doing their work and you will be setting yourself up for undigested foods moving on in the digestive track and improper digestion of the next meal.

Quality water is important to cleanse your digestive system before a meal and to keep your digestive organs properly hydrated so that they can do their work. The old tradition of a cup of thin soup before a meal helps with this process. We seldom take the time to do this any more, but it still is a good idea to hydrate the system about a half hour before a meal and to avoid cold drinks which will slow down digestion. Room temperature or lukewarm is best.

Within a week or two you are likely to sleep better, be more regular, and make wiser choices about eating without even thinking about it. And you will feel more interested in physical activity, maybe a walk, or checking out that unused membership at the gym, or maybe going dancing, swimming, or hiking with friends. Don't feel you need to overdo the exercise. Just enjoy the knowledge that your digestive system is repairing and working its way back into working order.

CHAPTER 10
MORE ENERGY BY REBUILDING THE BLOOD

The next step is to help rebalance and cleanse the blood. This is most easily accomplished by eating greens. Many of the lettuces we eat today come from a long history of trying to make our foods look pure by breeding them to be white rather than deep colored. This started in Roman times among the privileged classes. But now we know that the deeper the color, the more nourishing the food. We can list all the good things that have been discovered associated with the color, but there will always be more good things to discover, because every plant we eat is almost as complicated as we are.

Many vitamins are associated with deep colors, like vitamins A, B, and C. Vitamins were named about a century ago when it was found that without these micronutrients in our food, we developed specific symptoms of their absence. But many more substances have been discovered since then that are also very helpful to get from your food. And more will be discovered.

Today phytonutrients and antioxidants are getting all the attention. But the more we separate individual nutrients from their foods of origin, the less beneficial the results. Our body has a wisdom which we can't reproduce and it makes best use of the whole food with all its associated nutrients in their original order, not as a chemical soup.

For example, antioxidants were known about over 30 years ago, yet at that time the medical world scoffed at the idea that free radicals were a major cause of degeneration and disease. Free radicals form when substances in the body are oxidized. They become chemically joined to an oxygen molecule, much like iron when it rusts. They are then highly reactive and can cause a kind of chain reaction which interferes with vital processes and slows everything down.

Thirty years ago, it was known the vitamins E and C and the mineral selenium could prevent this kind of oxidation. But now an unending list of important antioxidants from foods is continuing to be discovered. The more exotic the fruit, for example, and the less manipulated by modern breeding and farming techniques, the higher the antioxidant activity of the fruit. That's why kiwi, assai, makai, noni, and other exotic fruits have become popular one after another. The bottom line is to trust real foods to feed you, not chemicals, and find them in as traditional and natural a form as you can.

The best color for cleansing the blood is green. Green, leafy vegetables go a long way to rebalancing and cleansing the blood. There are many different theories about why this is true, but what matters to us here is that it is true. It may be because the molecule of hemoglobin which carries oxygen through the blood to the cells resembles the molecule of chlorophyll which picks up the energy from the sun in a plant. Or it may be that the chlorophyll has other properties which help the blood to normalize the balance of fat, sugar, water, proteins, and minerals. Much cardiovascular disease has to do with inflammation of the linings of the blood vessels, lesions in the artery walls, and stickiness of fat particles passing by which get caught in these lesions. Chlorophyll seems to have a beneficial effect on all these conditions.

A salad a day can certainly help. The darker the greens the better. And add other colors while you're at it, with orange carrots, yellow squash or peppers, purple lettuces, red tomatoes, and so on. Sprouts which you can purchase fresh or grow yourself are also great sources of greens, very rich in enzymes. Try alfalfa or chia seeds. Eat a handful of the fresh greens or add them to your raw salad.

But if making a salad or growing your own sprouts takes too much energy at this point in your weight loss efforts, it's easy to get started by eating supplements of green foods. The most popular are barley grass, chlorella, spirilina, and wheat grass. These supplements come in powder or capsule form. I prefer the powder. Dr. Hagiwara discovered the amazing qualities of young barley grass over forty years ago and considered it the most perfect food. It had the most diverse and complete enzyme activity of any food when it is picked at the right time and processed quickly without heat.

When supplementing with greens, choose organic whenever possible to avoid any pesticides, herbicides, or imbalanced fertilizers used in agriculture and to avoid any genetically modified species.

As with digestion, proper hydration is critical to the health of the blood. Every cell in the body, from bone cells to pancreatic cells and brain cells, rely on the concentrations of different substances in the blood to be in proper balance so that nutrients are pushed into the cells and toxins pulled out.

So again, pay attention to quality water which is properly mineralized, alkaline, and energized, so that it will be highly usable by the cells. Often when we feel run down, depressed, or sleepy or we feel we have lost our concentration, a glass of fresh, purified, alkaline water will energize us right away by making our blood and other fluids flow easily, as they should.

Once you have added cleansing greens to your foods and are drinking pure water, you are likely to feel more energy and a greater sense of well-being in days or even hours. When the blood is happy, you will be too. In weeks or even days, some of the numerical indicators in your blood will most likely be improving too. Blood glucose, triglycerides, cholesterol, and other readings will tend to move towards healthier levels. But most important for your weight, you will be feeling more energy, and this will lead naturally to all the good habits which will bring you into a healthier place.

So start eating greens every day. A teaspoon of powdered young organic barley grass in the morning is a fantastic way to start the day off right. Take it in organic orange juice, pineapple juice, or tomato or mixed vegetable juice. You won't even taste the green taste. Then eat it again before each meal or as a snack. It feels energizing and delicious, and satisfying too. And because of your improved energy and sense of well-being, all your lifestyle habits will naturally start to improve.

CHAPTER 11
MORE ENERGY FROM FRIENDLY MICROBES

Symbiosis and synergy. These are big words but helpful and simple concepts. Symbiosis is the process by which two very different living creatures help support each other's lifestyle and help each other survive. And synergy is the process by which two things create unexpected benefits when acting together. That's what the healthy bacteria in your gut do. Known most often as lactobacillus, because they live comfortably on milk products, these bacteria are essential to our over all health.

Once you are rebalancing your digestion with digestive aids and rebalancing your blood with quality greens, the third thing you will want to do is to restore healthy balance to your intestinal tract. Absorption of nutrients will be enhanced and total abdominal comfort will be improved by tending to the well-being of the helpful microbes that inhabit your lower gut.

Recent emphasis on yogurt, kefir, and other naturally fermented foods, like sauerkraut and traditional fermented drinks, all emphasize the value of "probiotics." The term refers to food substances which encourage the repopulation of your lower digestive tract with microbes which actually help with the digestion of our foods. These good microbes, also called beneficial bacteria or bioflora, produce many essential nutrients, like vitamins K, B-12, and other B-vitamins which we then reabsorb and use in our bodies. These microbes work synergistically with your digestion in a symbiotic relationship.

They help to bulk up the stool as well, which keeps elimination more regular. When these beneficial microbes are happy, our digestive processes are happy and vice versa.

We all have a variety of microbes in our guts from the time we are born. We pick them up from our mothers and if we are breastfed we eat substances that specifically encourage the growth of the more beneficial microbes.

A major player here is Lactoferrin, a complex molecule which is produced in mother's milk and helps to set up a healthy environment in the newborn's gut. Lactoferrin has now been extracted from cow's milk and purified and concentrated so that it can be obtained as a supplement. The scientist who has done the most research on its amazing properties is Dr. Narain Naidu, who has developed a specific Lactoferrin supplement distributed by independent consultants with the global wellness giant Nikken, Inc.

We generally have an assortment of not so good microbes there too, so the trick is to keep the good ones in the majority. This takes some care, because the bad ones generally need only a bit of sugar and some undigested materials, while the good ones need fiber, quality fatty acids, and vitamins. Unfortunately one of the first things that happens when your body is under stress is that the unhelpful microbes can get the upper hand. These are most often a variety of yeast called Candida. Candida can produce gas, discomfort, and irregular stools. It can also change the digestion environment and discourage proper digestive acid production. It can even cross the intestinal barrier to get into the blood and cause immunological effects and inflammation.

To combat this development, you will want to support the good microbes and discourage the bad ones.

The easiest way to discourage the bad ones is to not feed them any carbohydrates for a few days, or as few as possible for a while. Meanwhile, focus on re-inoculating yourself with good bacteria from the probiotic foods. Make sure these foods still have viable bacteria or they cannot help to increase your beneficial microbe population.

Stress, antibiotics, imbalanced metabolism, cortisone or hormone treatments, pregnancy, illness, and many medications can change the bioflora balance. This is one reason bowel habits can change so quickly with stress or illness. And with the stress of excess weight and low energy, the beneficial microbial population is often the first to suffer.

Without a healthy bioflora in the gut, digestion can be incomplete, and elimination can be slow and prone to toxicity. For reasons discussed in previous chapters, this will lead to poor function or overwork for numerous organs throughout the body. You will tend to lack energy and feel run down. With low energy, you can predict that will power, counting, exercise, good food choices, self-esteem, and all those good things that are supposed to help you to loss weight will go out the window.

Almost every healthy food can serve as a "prebiotic." Prebiotics are foods which help to set up the right environment for probiotics, the healthy microbes, to dominate. A good vitamin and mineral supplement and a quality fatty acid supplement will go a long way to supporting your own happy bacteria. Omega 3 fatty acids are particularly helpful, but make sure these come from a reputable source, not from over processed fish oils. It's best to choose plant sources like flaxseed.

By restoring the symbiotic relationship we are meant to have with the helpful microbes in our gut, you will find many benefits. Among them will be improved digestion, comfort, and better energy flow. This will in turn support your weight loss efforts.

With these three steps to support digestion, rebalance the blood, and restore balance in the lower gut, I expect you will be delighted with the diminishing size of your waistline and the increasing amount of mental and physical energy you are now beginning to experience.

CHAPTER 12
MORE ENERGY FROM REDUCING TOXINS

The next most important step to create the energy you need to achieve your ideal healthy weight is to help your body to continuously cleanse and detoxify itself. Imagine living in a pristine world such as existed a thousand years ago, with no pollution of air, water, soil, or food. Even then there were poisonous plants which would get us in trouble if we ate them. But assuming we avoided those, we would still need our bodies to be cleansing, healing, and detoxifying to get rid of stuff every day.

When we eat other plants and animals, there are parts left over that are useless to us and must be detoxified and eliminated. Over the millennia, our bodies have developed a multitude of complex processes, like digestion, blood transport, and cell metabolism, to transform the good stuff into building blocks, fuel, and other necessary substances. But the insoluble fibers and other substances which are of no use to us must be processed and released through elimination. If they stay in the bowel or can't be properly processed by the liver, the immune system, and the kidneys, they will compromise the body's normal functions by interfering with the thousands of chemical reactions which must occur in our bodies every second.

In addition to the extras we must eliminate in the best of foods we eat, we must also eliminate the toxins which are the result of our normal bodily processes. We exhale the carbon dioxide which is a result of energy production. We must eliminate or neutralize all the acids which form from the cellular processes of building, repairing, and breaking down. We must detoxify the free radicals which are forming all the time from muscle action and other functions. And old enzymes, hormones, and cellular tissues which have outworn their usefulness must be broken down and disposed of.

To these natural detox challenges, from our food and our own internal activities, we must now add to the list all the toxins in our modern environment. There is an amazing amount of clean up to do and our bodies aren't set up for all these extras, so it helps to minimize the extra challenges whenever and wherever we can. And we must also protect and support our overworked detox and immune systems.

In the last few hundred years we have added all the by-products of industry, such as coal, and coal tars, oil and oil by-products, and the by-products of steel production and mining. Then in the last century we have added all the miracles of modern chemistry, including medicines derived from petrochemicals, lab-created vitamins, effluent into the air from power plants, fluoride in the water from aluminum production, pesticides and herbicides on our fields, household cleaners and disinfectants, personal care and cosmetic products, medical waste, radioactive waste, manipulated gene combinations for plants and animals which never occurred on the planet before, plastics, fire retardants, and more.

Just to take one example, a gene was discovered in the late 1990's in certain soil bacteria which has the ability to kill insect larvae by destroying their stomachs. Called Bt, this gene has been added to the genetic make-up of the U.S. corn crop and is now found in 65% of the crop. Recent evidence shows that this gene is found in the blood of over 67% of women and 80% of newborns. It has also been found to bind with the small intestine lining of mice and laboratory monkeys. This means it could become a serious toxin in our own digestive tracts. According to the EPA, the Bt proteins "Could act as antigenic and allergenic sources." This could mean trouble.

All such things are foreign substances to our bodies, not part of our bodies and not a normal part of our food or natural environments. They each act as a drag on our natural physiological processes. Together they form a toxic load which can sabotage our healthy energy output. Our bodies must recognize them as foreign and then deal with them as best they can. All of this is excessively demanding of our immune systems and our detox and elimination systems. Is it any wonder we are discovering so many new diseases of the bowel, the kidneys, the liver, the immune system, the lymph system, and the breathing organs?

The bottom line of a system which is overloaded with waste is the same as a home which has accumulated too much junk. Everything slows down. Energy is in short supply. Too much cellular energy goes into just trying to keep the waste and toxins at bay. Energy for feeling good, being active, being alert, and getting restful, restorative sleep is in short supply. We reach for something, anything, which will make us feel alive and kicking again.

What are some simple easy ways to clear house and make it easier for our bodies to focus on energizing us rather than just keeping basic functions free of sabotage from toxins and waste?

Here is where we talk about what to avoid. But again the trick isn't to try to change your eating habits dramatically just now while you still don't have the energy you need to feel like doing so. Instead we will start with making life easier for your body by reducing the total toxic load from all sources.

Stick with your favorite foods, but try to get them in a more natural form. Check labels to avoid added "preservatives, colorings, and artificial flavorings." Avoid artificial sweeteners, even the ones which call themselves natural, like "sucrolose." Though derived from a natural food, sucrolose has been so processed that your body cannot use it and will have to deal with it as a toxin. Avoid foods whose ingredient lists include chemicals you can't pronounce, unless they are added vitamins, in which case they will usually make that clear.

Lots of favorite foods now have more natural versions, since marketers know that consumers now feel "natural" is better. "Organic" is even better, since there are specific standards for organic, but not for natural. Organic foods, for example, are not allowed to include genetically modified organisms, GMOs.

Organic foods also must be free of antibiotics. Antibiotics are fed to most of the animals we raise for food and remain in the meat and the milk when we consume them. The antibiotics are used to help minimize the spread of disease among the severely overcrowded animals and to speed up growth and milk output. They are unnecessary if the animals are raised in a healthy, spacious environment. This means we must pay a bit more for organic meat and milk, but it's worth it. The antibiotics we eat this way are making it ever harder for us to maintain healthy bioflora in our intestines as well as setting things up for the emergence of super bugs. These super bugs are resistant to antibiotics and are now wreaking havoc in many hospitals.

Don't get hung up on these problems with our food supply. The worst offenders are easy to get rid of. Colorings, preservatives, and additives just cover up poor flavor or quality. Simply go for the products equivalent to the products you love which have fewer of these foreign substances and buy organic whenever you can.

Next, survey the chemicals you use in your house and switch to more natural versions. Many you may not even need once you think about it. Most important are your personal care products, because you are putting these directly on your skin. It is astonishing how many substances foreign to the body are in personal care products today. Most have never been thoroughly tested for their toxic effects. Even if by themselves they wouldn't bother most people, with all the other toxins we're exposed to, you never know if they may just be the last straw for you. Many people have skin problems which could go away with less exposure to some of these chemicals. Yet often we are led to buy more products with other chemicals hoping to deal with these problems.

Lead in lipstick, aluminum in antiperspirants, parabens in underarm products, all of these are known and serious toxins. Industry claims that links to neurotoxicity, dementia, and cancer, respectively, can't be proven. They also claim unconvincingly that the amounts are too small to matter, or that they aren't absorbed into the skin. But then how do nicotine and hormone patches work? It doesn't make sense to say the patches work but other chemicals are not absorbed. And what about the total toxic load? Can we afford to be exposed to yet another unnecessary chemical? And what about the population studies which show that those with neurological problems have higher than usual lead in their systems, that Alzheimer patients have a higher load of aluminum, and that virtually all breast cancer patients have parabens in their breast tissue?

Start reducing your toxic load just by starting to reduce how many toxins you put on your skin. As you clean up your digestion, body odors will likely reduce, and you won't need much deodorant and perfume. Likewise, your skin will become healthier and you will need less aggressive skin care and fewer cosmetics. Meanwhile, as these items need replacing, do a little homework and buy products with ingredients you have heard of or can pronounce. And don't be fooled by personal care products which say "made with" natural ingredients like flowers, or herbs, or whatever they think you will think is desirable. The product can be made with all kinds of other things too that you don't want on your skin.

Many people are concerned about having a "clean" house, but "disinfected" doesn't mean clean. The dirt from your yard may be a lot cleaner than the toxic chemical you may have just dusted or polished your floor with. And all these chemicals give off toxins into the air. So you are breathing them into your lungs without even realizing it, and that means into your body and blood. A little extra amount of simple glycerin soap can do just as well as a powerful detergent with a little extra scrubbing on your part to remove grime. Many brands with far less toxicity are now available for washing clothes and dishes which do just as well as the more powerful chemicals. Don't feel that everything must kill all the bugs. Nature wastes nothing. There will be invisible life on any surface anywhere within hours of laying down some toxic substance. The idea is not to breed superbugs by constantly killing off the weaker ones. Let the ones we can live comfortably with just be.

If you wash with lots of water and natural soaps that don't totally wipe out all our ordinary microbial co-inhabitants, odors in your home shouldn't be a problem. So avoid air fresheners. They are one of the newest and most insidious and dangerous additions to our homes, increasing allergies, asthma symptoms, headaches, rashes, and that run-down feeling which sabotages your efforts to be healthy and slim.

We can get upset about all the pollution from industry and we need to make our voices heard. But meanwhile there is more than most people think that we all can do in our own homes to reduce our toxic load. Yes, there is pollution we can't control coming into our homes in the air and in the water, but if we get a good water filter and a good air filter for our home, we are protecting ourselves and our families, reducing our toxic load, and increasing our health and energy at the same time. These products do not have to be expensive. Get devices which work right where you need them, for example, an air unit in the bedroom, and a water unit where the family gets their drinking and cooking water. You don't need to be purifying rooms you don't use much or water you use to wash the floor.

As with digestion and the blood, quality water is also a great help to your detox and elimination systems. Toxins must be diluted to be moved through the body and removed successfully. But too much acidic water can be an extra burden on your kidneys, so make sure your water is alkaline and of high quality so that it will be absorbed by the cells rather than just flushed through to be eliminated by the kidneys. Also, consider that much quality water can come from fresh fruits and vegetables. Here the water is already purified and energized by the plants.

Finally, try switching to more natural materials for your clothes, your bedding, your bathroom tissue, and even your furniture, floorings, and curtains, as these come to need replacing. Again don't feel you must be fanatical. This would just add more stress and rob you of energy. Do the simple things first, like throwing out air fresheners and replacing perfumed tissue, dish soap, and clothes detergent. You will begin to notice a difference in how you feel.

Now that you are reducing your overall toxic load, let's do some things to help improve your immunity and detoxification systems, another way to free energy to be used to help you feel good and achieve your best weight. First, take a good mineral supplement which includes not only the major minerals you need, like calcium and magnesium, but also the trace minerals your body uses, like zinc, selenium, and boron. Kelp and other sea vegetables are also a great natural source of a balanced mixture of trace minerals. The mineral magnesium is particularly cleansing and important in the cellular energy production processes. It also helps to relax muscles and helps to keep the cardiovascular system well balanced. It has been known for generations to help move along the action in a compacted bowel.

Go easy on your liver. Add fresh squeezed lemon or lime juice to your water. Use high quality olive oil and natural vinegar (not distilled) on your salads. Drink a glass of pure water a half hour before each meal. Keep alcohol intake modest, no more than one or two glasses (of modest size!) of wine or beer or one serving of liquor a day. Enjoy gentle herb teas if they are to your liking, like chamomile, green tea, milk thistle, red clover, sarsaparilla, and so on. Use stevia to sweeten to taste (stevia can be purchased in green packets to replace the aspartame and other undesirable sweetener packets).

Breathing is a great way to rebalance your body, expel gaseous toxins, and increase your energy. If you are feeling down, exhale completely and let the new air come in naturally. Then exhale completely again. Do this ten or eleven times and your energy will pick up. More oxygen to the brain and fewer toxins in the lungs and blood mean more energy and good feelings for you.

Don't underestimate the work your body does for you that you aren't even conscious of. It is an unfortunate fact of modern life that functions which once could be taken for granted now must be consciously protected and supported because of the polluted modern environment. But don't get discouraged. Take some small steps each week and feel encouraged by the changes you perceive as your energy level builds day by day.

CHAPTER 13
MORE ENERGY FROM KNOWING WHEN TO EAT WHAT

Earlier I mentioned how we all tend to put weight on in the belly area no matter what body type we are. But there are basically four different body types which have been recognized for over 2500 years, and they have a great deal to do with how much energy we feel in our bodies and our minds. My book *The Four Temperaments: A Rediscovery of the Ancient Way to Understand Health and Character* explores these types in great detail. It explains how they impact not only health and weight but also relationships, moods, personality, disease patterns, lifestyle habits, and career choices. But here we need only look at their effects on our energy production.

When you eat and what you eat when will affect how energetic you feel throughout the day, and different patterns affect different people differently depending on their body type. How energetic you feel affects how much you eat and the quality of your food choices. Knowing when to eat what depending on you body type can make all the difference in your weight loss success. So let's take a look at these effects.

It is relatively easy to determine your body type if you are overweight, because each of the four types has a distinctive distribution of excess fat. The ancient doctors thought the four types were differentiated by the proportions, balance and flow of what they called "humors," "fluids," or "airs." This balance determined your "temperament."

Today we know that these four types are largely determined by the particular hormonal gland system which your body tends to rely on most when in need of more energy. The ancients weren't totally wrong to imagine fluids balancing the body as they worked together. Hormones flow through the whole body and work together, sometimes one turning off as others turn on and sometimes working at the same time, to balance an amazing number of functions.

There are four major hormonal systems which affect our energy level, and when we are under stress, we tend to look to one or the other depending on our body type. This tendency starts from a very young age since it has a strong genetic component. Usually one or the other of your parents is the same type as you are.

When you are under stress, it makes no difference if the stress is happy or sad. It may be the stress of a tough day at work or the stress of a fun visit with a grandchild. In either case, you will tend to rely on your thyroid gland, your pituitary gland, your adrenal glands, or your sex glands to give you the energy boost you need. The one you rely on can be called your dominant gland or hormone system.

The most common pattern for those frustrated by their weight is the one dominated by the thyroid gland. This is the most common for three reasons. These people really prefer to be thin so they are eager to seek out weight loss programs. They also have very changeable moods and frustration is very common. The thyroid gland can change their energy level very quickly and the ups and downs can be particularly frustrating. They want a change. And in addition, when people of the other three types have exhausted their own dominant glands, the thyroid is the fall back energy producer.

The people of this type correspond to the ancient type called "melancholic." They put on weight in their tummies, sides of the hips, backs of the arms, and for women, the breasts. Sugar and caffeine are the most effective stimulants for the thyroid, so most people who have trouble losing weight are trying to get more energy by eating more carbohydrates, caffeine, or other stimulants to get their thyroid gland to turn up the boilers in the cells. Many people know they crave sugar but don't realize that this energy boost is also their downfall.

Using caffeine can be a temporary fix. It is free of calories if it's black coffee or diet soda, but it can only make the problem worse because it overtaxes the thyroid and puts you on an energy roller coaster which can eventually lead to hypoglycemia or diabetes, not weight loss.

A person of the second body type is the one which relies on the sex glands when in stress. She puts on her weight primarily in her buttocks. Waist and upper body stay relatively thin, as does the face, but thighs and butt store fat easily. Women in this group often complain that even when they put on weight, their breasts do not. This group corresponds to the ancient category called "sanguine." Obviously the sex glands can increase our energy output, since that is exactly what they do with romantic arousal. People of this type use fatty, creamy foods like butter, eggs, shellfish, cream cheese, and so on to stimulate the sex glands. They also like eastern type spices like cinnamon and curry, which are traditionally known for their aphrodisiac effects. These people like to be most active in the evening and tend to overeat then.

The third body type tends to put on extra weight above the waist. Their hips and legs stay thin, but their shoulders can become massive. In women the breasts can enlarge greatly with added weight. People of this type correspond to the ancient group called "choleric." They are governed by the adrenal glands, each of which sits atop a kidney. The adrenals are well known as the fight or flight glands. They go into action when we feel fear or, more commonly today, stress. As far as the body is concerned, stress is the same as fear. The adrenals get stimulated by proteins and salt, so people with this tendency are likely to match the "meat and potatoes" profile. They will go for a second hamburger rather than the ice cream or chocolate cake. They are very active throughout the day but usually crash early in the evening.

The fourth body type tends to accumulate weight fairly evenly all over, even in the face, so they stay youthful looking, and it is hard to guess their age. They often complain of fat knees since the other three types don't add much fat to their knees. These folks correspond to the ancient type called "phlegmatic." They rely most on the pituitary gland, which is known as the master gland. It regulates overall growth, but these people tend to be smaller rather than larger in frame. They usually like milk products best, since cow's milk has pituitary stimulating hormones in it. So milk gives them a bit of a pick me up. They also like berries and mild sweets, which resemble milk in their slightly sweet flavor. They usually don't like strong flavors of any kind. People of this temperament prefer to snack rather than eat big meals. They complain about sluggish metabolisms when dieting because they have usually increased their intake of cottage cheese or other milk products and have overwhelmed their pituitary gland.

For each of these temperaments, the important thing for losing weight is to eat the right things at the right time of day and avoid the wrong things at the wrong time of day. This simple approach will help you achieve steady energy output throughout the day, resulting in a stronger sense of well-being and a gradual, healthy return to healthy weight.

The melancholic person who wants to lose weight needs to have a hearty protein rich breakfast. Usually, in contrast, she will tend to have a light carbohydrate laden breakfast with a bit of caffeine. This sets her up to crave sugar or some stimulant about every two hours throughout the day, not a good pattern for losing weight. This is especially true if you are at work, where healthy, satisfying snacks during the workday are rare. Lunch and dinner also need to have a good portion of protein, along with some good quality fat. These help balance the thyroid output rather than keep it on a carbohydrate roller coaster.

Melancholic folks are often the first to go vegetarian, because they are highly principled people and don't like red meat much anyhow. But they need to avoid the high carb diet which many vegetarians are prone to. They also need to get regular protein and fat from eggs, beans, cheese, chicken and turkey; olives, nuts and seeds. They usually enjoy salads, so they can make it a habit to add these proteins to their salads.

If you eat this way as a melancholic type, you will naturally shift your energy level to being more consistent. Junk foods and sweet or starchy foods will lose their irresistible appeal. You can still enjoy your favorite foods, but only as part of a balanced meal and in just enough quantity to satisfy your desire for the flavor or texture. Snacks need to be from the non-carb categories, like vegetables with peanut butter, or a small handful of nuts. With your thyroid and energy output more balanced, your digestion will improve, your sleep will improve, and your shape and weight will move towards your ideal relatively effortlessly.

If you are of the sanguine type, you may be just the opposite of the melancholic. Not that you should load up on carbs, but rather, you need to have a smaller breakfast and be careful at what time of day you eat your fatty, creamy, or spiced things. Have a light breakfast with just a bit of protein and fat and some carbs. For instance, a nice bowl of granola or muesli (the traditional Swiss breakfast cereal of ground oats, nuts and fruits) will start your day off right. If you consume a predominantly fatty breakfast, like a large cheese omelet, you have stimulated your sex glands too early in the day and you may feel like eating too much for the rest of the day and even into the next day.

Ideally lunch would be your biggest meal, though this is hard to do as an employee on the job. At least keep lunch well balanced, like a salad with a small piece of fish or an egg. Dinner needs to be well balanced as well. You can still enjoy your favorite foods, but as with all types, they must be eaten with a balanced meal and not as your snacks. For the sanguine person, avoid fatty, creamy snacks like a handful of nuts or rich cheese. Instead have a few crackers or cold vegetables or a piece of fruit. And most important, do not eat late at night. If you do, you will be wanting more all the next day.

If you are of the choleric type, the same breakfast recommendations apply as for the sanguine. You will have to forgo the manly breakfast for a more modest, balanced meal. It's better to save the meats and omelets for later in the day. Otherwise the high protein and salts will over stimulate your adrenal glands and you will be exhausted early in the afternoon and want to eat more than you would otherwise during the rest of the day. Choleric folks aren't big on salad or vegetables, but these will help to balance out the adrenal glands and help to nourish the other glands and the whole body. So do your best to add them to your plate. Again you don't have to give up your favorite foods. Just eat them at the right time of day and with a balanced plate. Don't splurge at the end of the day with meat and salty snacks or you will have trouble sleeping and be tired and wanting more food the next day.

If you tend to be choleric, be sure to notice when you are thirsty, rather than taking extra salt to force you to drink fluids. People of the choleric type are the last to consider becoming vegetarian, but if they add a bit of butter and salt to their veggies, they will take to them more easily. Counting calories won't be half as effective as adding vegetables and fruits to the mix. People of this type rarely snack, but if they do, a glass of water or an apple would be best.

If you are of the phlegmatic type, your breakfast should not rely heavily on milk. Phlegmatic folks don't usually like eggs, so that's not likely to appeal to you for breakfast. But a bowl of granola with almond milk instead of cow's milk may be agreeable. Or substitute goat milk, which has much less pituitary stimulating hormone, since goats don't have to grow as big and fast as cattle. A heartier breakfast will serve you well too. A slice of no-nitrate ham on a piece of toast could be perfect. Or try a bowl of oatmeal with goat milk and raisins. Milk early in the day will cause your pituitary to dominate the day from the start. Again we are looking for balanced stimulation of all the glands and nourishment of the whole body and all its organs and systems, with the end goal of steady energy throughout the day.

It may seem that the melancholic dominant people and phlegmatic dominant people should eat most alike and the choleric people and sanguine people would do best to pair up at mealtime. But this is rarely what happens. Instead, melancholic people and sanguine people are most attracted to each other and the choleric people and phlegmatic people are most drawn together. This is because their personalities tend to complement each other best in these combinations. So when these pairs eat together, they need to know that they need to have a balanced meal before them, but then each is individually responsible to pick the foods and the portions that will suit them best to maximize steady energy throughout their day. Then if they get together again in the evening, they both will be in a much better mood than if they ate wrong for their type during the day, and they will get along much better. They will be feeling good about themselves and still have the energy they need to be good to themselves and their loved ones.

Those of the sanguine and choleric types tend to metabolize fats faster and more effectively than those of the melancholic and phlegmatic types. The latter tend to rely more on the carbohydrates for energy. Meanwhile, the choleric and melancholic types tend to have faster metabolisms than the sanguine and phlegmatic types. So you can see that your dominant tendency can make a real difference in how changes in your lifestyle can affect your weight loss success. This is one reason there are so many diet plans out there vying for your dollar. It is the lucky dieter who happens upon the right kind of diet for her body type.

The true secret is to know yourself and how you can personally adjust your thinking and your habits to create the energy you need to feel vibrantly healthy and eager for life.

CHAPTER 14
MORE ENERGY FROM SLEEP

We live in a sleep deprived nation. In times of economic growth, folks are running after their dreams. In times of economic slump, they are just running to keep up. Unfortunately the gap between the super rich and the modestly poor is growing ever wider and the latter supports the former. What they have in common is not enough sleep.

Every mammal ever studied and lots of other animal groups need a certain amount of sleep to thrive. Before the light bulb, we had only campfires, fireplaces, gas lamps, and candles to keep us awake after dark. Now people don't even expect to slow down when the sun goes down. But recent studies are piling up day after day showing that not enough sleep and interrupted or uncomfortable sleep are directly related to weight problems.

Certainly excess weight can cause poor sleep because of not finding a comfortable resting position, the closing off of the breathing passages causing snoring or the interrupted breathing of apnea, or discomfort from indigestion or poor elimination. But it is also true that poor sleep quantity and quality can contribute to causing a person to accumulate extra weight.

Scientists have theorized a number of reasons for the connection. They know for example, that the hormone leptin is rebuilt primarily at night during a deep sleep. Leptin helps to tell us when we are satisfied with the quantity of food we have eaten. Also, inadequate sleep is treated as a stress by the body, so our stress reactions go into overtime when we don't sleep enough. The hormone cortisol, which is the stress hormone which puts fat around our middle, increases with lack of sleep. And the immune system, which is responsible for recognizing toxins and steering them to the right handler organ, becomes severely depressed with not enough sleep, even after one night.

Many people know they are feeling run down and vulnerable to the current cold or flu microbes when they have pulled an all-nighter for work or have tossed and turned all night. That's the immune system overloaded and unable to do its job. A recent study found that people who did not keep the same waking and sleeping hours from weekday to weekend actually suffered what the researchers said was equivalent to jet lag. Their natural body rhythm was distorted and they felt rundown and uneasy much of the week.

Scientists in Japan have also found that the natural magnetic energy of the earth has a powerful relaxation effect on the body. Today our sleep environments cut us off from this natural source of calm. Almost all our houses and buildings where we sleep are on concrete slabs which block the earth's calming energy. It is no wonder we go to the mountains, the beach, or the forest to relax and rejuvenate. Our bodies love that clean air, the beneficial negative ions in the air, and the calming surroundings. But it is also the magnetic energy from the ground which refreshes and relaxes us.

A visionary company in Japan, Nikken, Inc., was the first to develop a sleep pad which incorporated natural rare earth permanent static magnets into the sleep surface to replicate that powerful relaxation effect. It is still the leader in this technology. Surrounding the body with an earth-like magnetic field is actually the only known way to facilitate the deepest stage of the natural sleep cycle. No sleep medication so far developed can do that. In fact, the sleep medications drug the brain. They do not put it to sleep.

It is when in a deep sleep that your memory sorts out the impressions of the day, your muscles relax and rebuild, your immune system reboots, and your digestion rebuilds. Without four or five repetitions of the full 90 minute sleep cycle without waking up, we cannot be at our best. So it is important we be as comfortable as possible so we don't need to interrupt these cycles to get more comfortable.

Sleeplessness is a huge stress on our bodies. Chronic inadequate time asleep or interrupted sleep has been associated with many cognitive and health problems. Even just three nights without sleep is considered abject torture and leads to hallucinations, failed judgment, disorientation, and even insanity. It is a frightening fact that today as many car accidents occur as a result of sleep deprivation as occur because of driving under the influence of alcohol or drugs.

Are we getting fat because we are sleepy? Are we eating to stay awake? These things just might be true. If they may be for you, let's see what changes you can make.

First, go to bed close to the same time every night and plan on waking up at least seven or eight hours later. A recent study busted the myth that we sleep less and less well as we age. After interviewing a large number of elderly people, the researchers found that these people tended to feel content with their sleep. So don't use the excuse that you need less sleep now or that your age makes you sleep less well.

For many, work schedules make it essential to do some catching up on weekends, but minimize the difference as much as possible. And studies have shown that catching up really isn't very effective when it comes to immune suppression, energy production, and mood.

If you tell yourself you will sleep better, it will help to reset your expectations. Many people get into a vicious cycle, assuming they will have a tough night and they do. They may have trouble falling asleep, or wake up after a few hours to go to the rest room or get a snack, or have trouble returning to sleep, or wake up in early morning restless but still exhausted. Some get into the habit of assuming that some time during the night they will need a sleep medication. The reason labels on these medications instruct not to take them if you must be active, drive, or operate dangerous machinery within eight hours is because they interfere with your perception and memory. Don't be fooled into thinking they will just help you sleep for those eight hours. You will indeed be mentally impaired for those eight hours. If you use sleep pills, they are another toxin your body must expend energy to recover from. Try to wean from them as soon as you can.

Check your bedtime routine. Don't watch scary movies or disturbing news and don't play angry video games right before bed. Don't eat stimulating foods, especially those that stimulate your dominant gland, within two hours of your bedtime. Enjoy some quiet reading or watch a favorite fun movie or comedy show instead. Drink a little pure water and brush your teeth with natural toothpaste. Make sure the temperature and humidity of your room is comfortable. See that the room is completely dark near your bed or wear a sleep mask. Make sure it is quiet.

If you don't have a magnetic sleep pad as described above, then make it a habit to step outside a little before bedtime. Step off the concrete and onto the ground and suck up the soothing magnetic power of mother earth. Breathe deeply, close your eyes, and be thankful for your growing health and energy.

When you are regularly sleeping long enough and deep enough, you will start to wake up more refreshed, flexible, looking good, and eager to get moving. Your mornings will once again be something to look forward to, like when you were a little kid. Believe you can get back that kind of energy and feel good, good about yourself and good about your improving health and weight control.

CHAPTER 15
MORE ENERGY FROM PLATE AND PORTIONS

Now that you have a good idea of how to time your foods to help keep your energy flowing, let's take a look at your plate. I mentioned a balanced meal. The prevailing idea of what a balanced meal is has shifted dramatically over the last fifty years. When I was a child, it basically meant some meat, some vegetables, some grain or root vegetable, and a salad, with a sweet dessert to finish it off and a glass of water to help "wash it down." Since then we have been through the high protein diet, the Hollywood diet, the low carb diet, the whole grains diet, the drinking man's diet, the macrobiotic diet, the fermented diet, the vegetarian diet, the Mediterranean diet, the South Beach diet, the fruitarian diet, the raw foods diet, the food combination diet, the locavore diet, and even the grapefruit diet.

Both the best and the worst thing about human eating capacity is that we can eat just about anything which won't kill us right away. We have inherited the earth because we can live entirely on fruit and nuts that fall from trees year round in the tropics, or we can live on seal muscle, blubber, and entrails for an entire winter until a few greens appear in the arctic spring.

That's a plus, to be able to adapt so well to whatever is edible in our region. Many of our ethnic ancestors acclimatized to certain diets and we would do well to pay attention to our dietary heritage.

But it's a negative that we can do so well on denatured, fractionated, concentrated, extracted, manipulated, purified, and otherwise altered foods. This is where the diseases of modern civilization come from, and they are spreading around the world as cultures adopt our over fabricated diet. This phenomenon was identified, investigated, and documented many years ago, most notably by T.L. Cleave of the British Royal Navy, and by Weston A. Price.

I saw this progression myself in my three visits to the Tahitian Islands in French Polynesia in the South Pacific. My visits spanned just under 10 years and in that time I saw the children change from all looking healthy and acting happy to being a mixture of too fat and too skinny and to being argumentative and sullen. In the holds of our cruise ships we discovered that we were delivering to these islands ever more processed foods from the U.S. They were taking their toll, most notably on the children.

So what is a balanced plate today? It can be said that it's best to decide ahead of time whether you are focusing on protein or carbs in each meal. If you have equal quantities of both, your stomach won't know quite what to do. But even this mild suggestion is unnecessary if you are dedicated to thoroughly chewing your food.

The stomach interprets what responses your mouth is giving to the food you are chewing and "decides" from that what juices it needs to produce. Really all you need to do is think of making the food on the plate have a variety of color, be not too big, and have proteins, carbs, and fats in the proper proportions for your body type and the time of day.

A good rule of thumb for what your stomach can actually handle comfortably is to eat no more at one sitting than is the equivalent of your two fists brought together at the wrists. If you are a little woman, your hands are small and if you are a big man, your hands are big. This way your body can tell you how much to eat without any counting.

And you don't have to worry about fat calories versus carb calories if you are attending to your particular body shape. Fat packs more calories per gram than sugars and carbs, but it is also more satisfying if you eat slowly enough to notice. So you will tend to eat fewer fat grams than carb grams, unless you are eating mindlessly and not noticing what or how much is going down or how you are feeling.

Remember, if we didn't enjoy eating, we would quickly perish. Gathering together to eat is a defining characteristic of the human species. So plan on taking time to choose your food, prepare it, share it, and enjoy it, free of regret and guilt. You are transforming the energy of other life forms into energy for your own life. Make it a good experience each time.

Isn't that a lot easier than counting and measuring every bit of food you plan to eat or analyzing your food to death? Once we have attended to digestion, blood, detox, body shape, and sleep, plate and portion control become an enjoyable right brain activity, meant to be enjoyed as the life affirming transformational energy process it is.

If you suffer from allergies to various foods or get reactions to gluten or other food components, do not assume this is a permanent state. As your digestion, blood, and detox systems become less burdened and healthier, your body may heal itself to such an extent that these foods may not cause a problem any more.

A word here about soy. Many people have heard good things about soy, especially that it is a staple in Asia where many people stay thin and healthy. But the way soy is processed here and used in every kind of food to mimic all kinds of textures and flavors has caused concern about its effects. In Asia time honored processing and fermentation have eliminated unwanted aspects of soy. But modern commercial processing tends to skip these steps. Many people who are trying to lose weight find that they do better avoiding soy. Some research suggests it can interfere with thyroid function and other hormonal processes. Also, most of the soy used in this country is genetically modified, and the effects are still completely unknown. I prefer not to be the guinea pig for new foods no human body has ever known before.

Many worry that when they are at work or on the go with kids or grandkids or attending to service projects, they cannot make the food choices they wish they could. There is a simple answer here. Now there are some truly high quality meal replacement powders which are free of all objectionable ingredients and they taste good too. Find a meal powder which is not a pure protein powder or designed for high performance athletes, just one which gives you a complete meal. A new source of easy to digest protein is a special

French pea, used in the Kenzen Body Balance powder from Nikken, Inc.

Choose formulations which are free of added salt, artificial flavors, artificial sweeteners, and preservatives. It is also good to avoid gluten, lactose, and other diary, like casein or whey, if you are sensitive to these. And avoid GMOs whenever possible. If it doesn't say it is free of GMOs, then you can expect that it contains them. Try to find a powder which claims to support your bioflora as well, "prebiotic" or "probiotic."

Mixed with goat milk or almond milk or with purified water, these meal replacement powders make a complete and satisfying meal. But eat it slowly, because though it is in liquid form, it is an entire meal and you want your digestion to get the right signals to digest it properly. Take it in a thermos to keep it cold, shake, savor, and enjoy.

Some interesting recent research has shown that dieting is the worst thing for your weight. Not just the ups and downs of yo-yo dieting, but also the idea of depriving yourself when your body wants you to eat. The brain plays tricks on you when you deny its basic instinctual messages. If you feel like you need some energy input and you refuse to oblige, chances are very good you will feel deprived and overcompensate later. For example, one study found with diabetics that even if they use artificial sweeteners in drinks and other products, they will end up consuming just as much refined carbohydrate overall as if they didn't take the fake sweets. The body doesn't tolerate fraudulent food in the long run.

It may also be true that those who are dieting too hard may be actually eating too little rather than too much, or at all the wrong times, as we have seen. If the body detects that you are not eating when it tells you that you want to, it may decide you are under stress. It may start slowing down your metabolism to conserve energy and start storing fat away for the hard times to come.

Instead, you need to avoid imposing minute judgments on your every move with respect to food and begin to trust your body signals once you have begun to apply the steps outlined earlier. As you become more understanding of what your body is really telling you and really trying to do, knowing when, what, and how much to eat will become obvious to you in an ongoing comfortable way.

So instead of being on a "diet," think of a balanced plate as beginning with a bit of protein, like egg, cheese, beans, oatmeal, nuts, seeds, fish or meat. Then add a pile of vegetables, raw and cooked, of all different colors. Then add a bit of some grain or root vegetable, like a slice of whole wheat bread or a small potato. Finally include a bit of high quality fat, like a pat of fresh butter or a tablespoon of olive or peanut oil. Avoid oils which have been hydrogenated or chemically extracted. These have unhealthy trans fats and chemical residues.

The higher the quality of the basic ingredients, the better your meal will taste without a lot of seasonings, spices, sauces, or fancy preparation. And the simpler the food, the easier it is for your digestion to get a handle on what needs to be done. Use fruits as desserts or snacks or in small amounts as condiments.

When you plan your plate, use what I call my WOLFSPRING™ plan: Try to make the food on your plate as **W**hole, **O**rganic, **L**ocal, **F**resh, **S**imple, **P**ure, **R**aw, **I**n season, **N**ot irradiated, and **G**enetically traditional as possible. Stay tuned for my new book giving more detail about the WOLFSPRING™ plan.

Also, make the food on your plate as colorful as you can. If it is all shades of white and brown, your body will not be getting the variety of energies it requires. Add green, yellow, orange, red, blue, and purple.

Even a pizza can qualify as a balanced meal if the dough is organic and whole grain, the tomatoes are organic and local, the cheese is not processed and is free of antibiotics, and the oil is extra virgin olive oil. Such pizzas do exist, but you might have to search the frozen food section of your natural food store, find a vegetarian restaurant which specializes in healthy foods, or make them yourself. Just add a small salad, make sure the quantity of pizza is not too large for your stomach, and enjoy.

CHAPTER 16
MORE ENERGY FROM MOVEMENT

Okay, here we are recommending physical activity after saying it is not what makes you thin. That is still true. You are not nor have you ever been lazy. We saved this topic for late in the book because it is one of the last things that changes. When you don't have energy, you are not going to want to move much. It's that simple.

You may love hiking, biking, swimming, dancing, tennis, touring, or whatever. But if the energy isn't there, something more sedentary will hold more appeal. Don't feel bad. That's totally natural.

I have known people to go to the gym every day to try to burn off calories only to feel fatigued and discouraged with little weight loss for all that effort. Exercise can easily be overdone. Too much can cause inflammation, water retention, and real stress. New research is showing that there is a difference between health and what we think of as "fitness." Lots of athletes are on a roller coaster of manipulating their bodies for peak performance only to have slow and miserable recoveries. Overusing a muscle can be as dangerous as under using it and excessive exercise creates an amazing number of free radicals and acids which the body must detox and eliminate, using precious antioxidants and alkalizing minerals.

So don't feel your weight won't change unless you begin a strenuous exercise routine. In fact, be especially careful of machines which use numbers to say whether you are doing well or not. The machine doesn't know if you are building your internal torso muscles or straining your peripheral muscles, for example. Some more traditional trainers in yoga, calisthenics, and isometrics have noticed that some fitness programs make the mistake of distorting your muscle systems for specific results. You need to stay aware of the health of your whole body. Don't let a few favorite machines throw other muscle groups out of whack. Some overenthusiastic workout customers wind up with residual problems in back, neck, shoulder, or knee which eventually keep them from feeling like any exercise at all.

When you are beginning to be more active, stick with activities humans have always done. Remember, the first man who ran a marathon dropped dead when he delivered his message. Take a short walk down the street, stopping to smell the flowers or to watch the birds or the people. Sit or lie on the ground and stretch yourself gently in ways that feel good. Forget the "no pain no gain" that some trainers love. Your body knows best. Just plan on doing a bit more each day as your energy grows.

A vigorous daily walk has been a timeless recommendation by health experts for centuries. Movement creates energy if it is done within normal limits. The body has an amazing system, the lymph system, which draws toxins and waste away from every cell in your body, detoxes them in the lymph nodes, and sends the remains to the liver to be processed and eliminated. It does not have a pump like the blood system has in the heart. It is pumped only by general muscle movement throughout the body. So gentle movement has a direct effect on your detox system. It also improves digestion, since the use of the leg and abdominal muscles as in a good walk helps with the peristalsis, which is the internal muscle movement which aids in digestion.

If you have a rebounder (a mini-trampoline) in your home, a mild bouncing can improve lymph flow, digestion, well-being, and thus energy production. The same effect is achieved by dancing, swimming, and walking. Running on asphalt or concrete is a major strain. Find a nice gravel or grass track at your local park if you want to run, but keep it at a jog which is comfortable for you.

People worry about cardiovascular fitness, which it is assumed means you must raise your pulse past a certain level on a regular basis. Studies have shown that with a half hour brisk walk, swim, or jog you will do just as well for heart health as with a heavy-breathing run. Meanwhile you will have to deal with fewer free radicals and acids created and with less overall stress to the body. So take a half hour walk and forget feeling badly about not running for 10 minutes and checking your pulse all the time.

Trust your body to want to be fit and healthy and listen to it as you gradually increase your physical activity. Feel good about moving a little more because your brain and your body are starting to feel more like doing it. You are working with your precious body instead of against it now, and it will love you for it.

CHAPTER 17
MORE ENERGY FROM IMAGINATION

Much has been said about body image. Starved models on the runways and diet ads in every medium distort our imagination so we don't feel good about ourselves. As girls and boys try to look like their music video stars at younger and younger ages, we watch the sad commercialization of their precious power of imagination. Kids are famous for their great imaginations. We seem to lose our imaginations as we age. Now let's exercise the imagination muscle in our favor.

Picture yourself as you wish to be, wearing a great outfit or nothing at all and liking what you see in the mirror. Know that is who you are already. You may have let your imagination be polluted by misinformation about what you should look like or what makes you put on weight. Now you know the truth. The true secret is energy. We are all just sophisticated patterns of energy. The atoms we think of as creating matter are only concentrated bits of energy which are in the habit of behaving certain ways relative to each other. And your imagination uses energy too. Flex that muscle.

If you like, take out a sheet of paper and draw a line down the middle. On the left side of the page, write down all the sayings of misinformation you have listened to about your body, your weight, your shape, your hopes of achieving your ideal weight, and your dreams of being and looking your best.

Then opposite each saying on the paper, write down what you believe now. Repeat these new sayings over and over to yourself until they are what you hear in your mind whenever you hear the old sayings. You may still hear them from well meaning relatives or friends or see them or read them in diet ads. But now you can affirm in your head the real truth.

Say to yourself, "I am building my energy and I am radiating health through my body and to everything around me. Everything I eat adds to my energy and I easily discard all things that detract from my vibrant health."

Spell out something like that in your own words and repeat it morning and night. Write it out and decorate it artistically in any way that speaks to you. Hang it where you will see it often. Have faith that the universe and divine providence are on your side. You are meant to be healthy and happy and you are well on your way.

Our imaginations can add to our level of stress by imagining what can go wrong in any situation. We can feel bad about what has happened in the past, we can feel anxious about what might be happening now, and we can worry about the future. Our mere thoughts can add stress to our lives which can in turn cause us to feel run down and unable to do what we must do to regain and maintain our healthy weight.

It is sad news that over one third of women's visits to doctors' offices involve prescriptions for antidepressants and women receive twice as many antidepressant prescriptions as men, according to the National Center for Health Statistics. According to *Saving Women's Hearts*, by Dr. Martha Gulati and Sherry Torkos, antidepressants often have unwanted side effects including weight gain, as well as poor sleep, sexual dysfunction, and increased anxiety and stress.

Stress caused by our own mental imaginings is the kind of stress we can control. We can flex our imagination muscle to imagine good stuff happening. We can let go of bad feelings about the past, along with any guilt or regret, and instead know that we have the power to limit any bad consequences by what we do today. We can let go of anxiety about present circumstances and instead set our imaginations to finding out what we can do within our power today to improve things. And we can stop worrying and feeling fearful about the future and instead remind ourselves that the small choices we make today will add up to big rewards in the future.

When your imagination is leaning the wrong way, consider these simple steps: stop what you are doing and drink a glass of quality water; take a look out the window and enjoy a tree or the sky for a moment; play with your dog or cat for a few minutes; exhale slowly until you are moved to breathe in; chew a piece of fresh fruit, like half an apple, pear, or banana; or walk around the room smiling. Any of these steps are stress fighters. They will help to overcome your stress reactions and any depression or hopelessness you may feel. They free up your imagination for better things, so that your energy can be renewed.

It's easy to forget the power of choice which is ours every moment of the day. When you are feeling fatigued, run down, and short of energy the range of choice seems narrow. But if you start to make small changes in the direction of the suggestions in this book, you will have more of the energy you need to put your imagination to work to reduce your mental stress and to see a wider range of choices. In turn, your healthy imagination will help reduce feelings of stress, increase your ability to respond to your day in healthy ways, and help to restore your natural energy.

If a long list of things to do is getting you down and you just don't have the energy, again use your imagination. Picture the tasks already accomplished and then figure out what small steps you can take to accomplish the rest. Often when we take time to prioritize and to distinguish between things that seem urgent and things which are actually necessary, we can accomplish much more. If you take the time to garner energy from the power of your imagination, then all your energy restoring strategies will complement each other.

Affirm for yourself that the boulders which stood in the way of achieving your ideal weight have been removed. Have faith that your body is on your side and is not your enemy. It wants to be healthy and happy and to serve you through a long and satisfying life. Love it and it will treat you well. It will start telling you the truth about what you really want to eat, what you really want to do with your body, and how you really want to move through your day. It will tell you that you are now on track to have all the energy you need from now on to be clear of mind and sound of body.

CHAPTER 18
THE NEW ENERGIZED YOU

As you take the steps in this book, here is what can happen. First your waist reduces as your digestion improves. Then your skin, breathing, and elimination will get better. Sleep will be easier. Your moods will improve and you will notice you have more energy and fewer cravings. You will see that your food choices make more sense and your portion choices will be more in line with who you are becoming. You will feel more like being active with friends, walking, and even working. You will know that your body is working for you instead of against you. You will hear more compliments about how well you look. You will smile more, not just to be nice which you probably already do, but because you feel so good.

In the first week or two you will notice things are changing. In a month or two you will absolutely know you are finally on the right track. As you see the inches coming off and the pounds coming off, you will be thankful you have discovered the truth, that the true secret to weight loss is energy. You were never weak willed, lazy, gluttonous, or uncaring. You were simply misled by a culture which doesn't understand how the body works, how the mind works, and how they work together. Now you know how to build energy into your mind-body system and you will feel better and great, for the rest of your life.

When people ask what you're doing, don't tell them! Just smile and tell them to get this book!

ACKNOWLEDGMENTS

I have had many awesome mentors in my search to understand the workings of our miraculous bodies and how to best support them and keep them working happy and healthy for a lifetime. Chief among these have been Dr. Kenneth Fordham, Dr. Ross Hume Hall, Dr. Leonore Britt, Dr. Harold Buttram, Susan Silberstein, Scott and Helen Nearing, Dr. Jody Rubin Pinault, Dr. Roger Drummer, Dr. Narain Naidu, Angie Peacetree, Sally Fallon, Alice Baland, Jean Antonello, and Michio Kushi. To each I give my heartfelt thanks.

I wish also to thank my physician father, who instilled in me a deep trust of nature, and also my mother and her father, who showed me the joy of helping garden vegetables to grow naturally. I appreciate so much the many inspiring teachers in all the nutrition courses, workshops, and seminars I have attended. I also am grateful to the hundreds of mentors I have in print, in the books on health and nutrition I have devoured over the past forty years.

I want to thank all my clients, students, and audience participants, who have helped to expand my knowledge of what works best for real people. And finally I want to thank my husband, my son, and my daughter, who have always been willing to go along with my experiments, to encourage my study and teaching, and to trust me enough to ask for and often listen to my advice.

ABOUT THE AUTHOR

Randy Colton Rolfe is an author, speaker, mother, and grandmother, and world ambassador for family. She chose her life mission early as a result of traveling with her family in 29 countries before age 20, during 12 summers. She saw both the differences and common desires of all peoples and decided to find out what it took to make families happy and healthy.

She achieved top academic honors at the Shipley School in Bryn Mawr, PA, at the University of Pennsylvania (BA in International Relations), at Villanova Law School (Law Review Editorial and Administrative Board), and at Villanova University Graduate School (MA in Theology). She married her college sweetheart John Rolfe, also a lawyer, speaker, and author.

For several years Randy practiced litigation and corporate law with a top Philadelphia law firm (the first woman lawyer ever hired there). Then, declaring their independence from corporate America in 1976, she and John moved to rural upstate New York to homestead and to begin their family. They renovated a 135 year old farmhouse, minimized wiring to maximize natural energy in the home, heated and cooked with wood they had cut themselves, and ate from their organic garden.

There they enjoyed raising their son and daughter. Meanwhile they used their legal skills to help the local farmers and Native Americans fight the New York State Power Authority to preserve their land from the dangers of a new ultra high voltage transmission line.

Upon their return to Pennsylvania, Randy became certified in Applied Clinical Nutrition by the University of Pennsylvania Dental School. She then served as a nutrition educator for Nutri-Systems and for several natural health food stores. As an attorney, she helped to develop the legal foundation for what is now called emissions "cap and trade" for the City of Philadelphia Department of Air Quality Control. In 1985 she founded the Institute for Creative Solutions and gave hundreds of seminars, a number of college courses, and private counseling on nutrition, parenting, marriage, and family.

Randy became a sought after guest expert on hundreds of radio shows and over 50 major network TV talk shows, including 20 times on *Geraldo Rivera,* 6 times on *Sally Jessy Raphael*, and dozens more.

Even though she had been a chubby teenager, Randy became a winner in several beauty pageants, including Mrs. Pennsylvania 1993. For her volunteer work, Randy was awarded the Chapel of the Four Chaplain's Legion of Honor.

In 1997 Randy joined Nikken, Inc. as an independent consultant, adding Nikken's pioneering wellness and life balance solutions to her offerings to help families to thrive worldwide. You can partner with her as an independent Nikken consultant at www.nikken.com/randyrolfe.

Randy's most recent book is *Mothers Losing Mothers: Comfort and Reassurance in Your Time of Loss*. Randy's previously published books include:

You Can Postpone Anything But Love: Expanding Our Potential As Parents;

Adult Children Raising Children: Sparing Your Child From Co-Dependency Without Being Perfect Yourself; The Seven Secrets of Successful Parents;

The Four Temperaments: A Rediscovery of the Ancient Way of Understanding Health and Character;

The Affirmations Book for Sharing: Daily Meditations For Couples (with her husband John Rolfe);

Princess Buttercup The Cat's Cross-Country Road Trip #3 (with her husband John Rolfe); and

101 Great Ways to Improve Your Life, vol. 3 (with David Riklan, Ken Blanchard, and others.)

Randy hosts a weekly talk radio program online called *Family First* where she interviews a different expert each week on diverse aspects of family life. *Family First* airs live on Fridays at 1PM Pacific/ 2PM Mountain/ 3PM Central/ 4PM Eastern, on the VoiceAmerica Health & Wellness Channel. The program can be accessed live or on archive by logging on at http://www.voiceamerica.com/show/1916/family-first. All previous shows are available in Randy Rolfe's Content Library for your on-demand and pod cast download use at http://www.voiceamericahealth.com. To book Randy for a speaking presentation, please go to www.expertclick.com. Or you can visit her on Facebook.

You can get any of Randy's books through her website www.randyrolfe.com, on www.amazon.com, and in eBook format for Kindle from Amazon and for Nook from Barnes & Noble. You can also read them on your PC, MAC, iPad, iPhone, and Android by getting a free download of the Kindle app at www.amazon.com or of the Nook app at www.bn.com. Be sure to register for Randy's free weekly newsletter full of great information about nutrition, parenting, and family, at www.randyrolfe.com.

www.ingramcontent.com/pod-product-compliance
Lightning Source LLC
Chambersburg PA
CBHW020335290526
45785CB00005B/2030